EYE CANCER SURVIVAL

GUIDE

A comprehensive resource for patient and family

Chapter 1: Introduction

- Paragraph 1: Definition and overview of eye cancer

- Paragraph 2: Importance of early detection and treatment

- Paragraph 3: Purpose and scope of the book

Chapter 2: Types of Eye Cancer

- Paragraph 1: Retinoblastoma (definition, symptoms, diagnosis)

- Paragraph 2: Uveal melanoma (definition, symptoms, diagnosis)

- Paragraph 3: Other types of eye cancer (e.g., conjunctival melanoma, orbital tumors)

Chapter 3: Causes and Risk Factors

- Paragraph 1: Genetic factors (e.g., family history, inherited syndromes)

- Paragraph 2: Environmental factors (e.g., UV exposure, smoking)

- Paragraph 3: Other risk factors (e.g., age, ethnicity)

Chapter 4: Symptoms and Diagnosis

- Paragraph 1: Common symptoms (e.g., vision changes, eye pain)

- Paragraph 2: Diagnostic tests (e.g., imaging, biopsy)

- Paragraph 3: Importance of early detection

Chapter 5: Treatment Options

- Paragraph 1: Surgery (e.g., enucleation, tumor resection)

- Paragraph 2: Radiation therapy (e.g., external beam, brachytherapy)

- Paragraph 3: Other treatments (e.g., chemotherapy, immunotherapy)

Chapter 6: Case Studies and Patient Stories

- Paragraph 1: Personal accounts from patients with eye cancer

- Paragraph 2: Insights from medical professionals

- Paragraph 3: Lessons learned and takeaways

Chapter 7: Latest Research and Advancements

- Paragraph 1: Emerging treatments (e.g., gene therapy, nanotechnology)

- Paragraph 2: Current clinical trials and studies

- Paragraph 3: Future directions in eye cancer research

Chapter 8: Resources and Support

- Paragraph 1: Organizations and advocacy groups

- Paragraph 2: Online resources and support communities

- Paragraph 3: Financial and emotional support options

Chapter 1: Introduction.

"Eye cancer **refers to a group of malignant diseases that affect the eyes, including the eyelids, conjunctiva, uvea, retina, and optic nerve. It is a relatively rare condition, accounting for only about 1% of all cancer diagnoses. However, early detection and treatment are crucial, as eye cancer can be life-threatening and may result in vision loss or even blindness if left untreated.**"

"Detecting eye cancer early is crucial, as it can significantly improve treatment outcomes and save vision. In fact, if caught early, some eye cancers have a survival rate of over 90%! Unfortunately, many people don't notice symptoms until the disease has progressed, making treatment more challenging. That's why it's essential to be aware of the risks, recognize potential symptoms, and seek medical attention promptly if you notice anything unusual. By being proactive and informed, you can take charge of your eye health and potentially prevent vision loss or even save your life."

"This book is designed to empower you with knowledge and hope. Whether you're facing a diagnosis of eye cancer, supporting a loved one, or simply seeking to understand the condition, this book aims to guide you through the journey. We'll delve into the types of eye cancer, their causes and risk factors, symptoms, diagnosis, treatment options, and ways to cope with the emotional and practical aspects of the disease. Our goal is to provide clear, concise, and compassionate information, helping you make informed decisions and navigate the path ahead with confidence."

Types of Eye Cancer,

Retinoblastoma (definition, symptoms, diagnosis).

"Retinoblastoma is a rare childhood cancer that develops in the retina, the light-sensitive tissue at the back of the eye. It typically affects children under the age of five and is the most common primary eye cancer in children. Symptoms may include a white glow or cat's eye reflex in the pupil, crossed eyes or strabismus, and vision loss or blindness. Diagnosis typically involves a comprehensive eye exam, imaging tests like ultrasound or MRI, and genetic testing to identify any inherited genetic mutations. Early detection is crucial, as retinoblastoma can be treated effectively with surgery, chemotherapy, or radiation therapy if caught in its early stages."

Uveal melanoma (definition, symptoms, diagnosis).

"Uveal melanoma is a type of eye cancer that develops in the uvea, the middle layer of the eye. It is the most common primary eye cancer in adults and can occur in the choroid, ciliary body, or iris. Symptoms may include:

- Blurred vision or vision loss
- Floaters (spots or cobwebs in vision)

- Eye pain or discomfort

- Sensitivity to light

- Redness or swelling of the eye

- Change in eye color or shape

Diagnosing uveal melanoma typically involves:

- Comprehensive eye exam (ophthalmoscopy)

- Imaging tests like ultrasound, MRI, or CT scans

- Fluorescein angiography (a test that highlights blood vessels in the eye)

- Fine-needle biopsy (removing a small tissue sample for examination)

Early detection is crucial, as uveal melanoma can spread to other parts of the body if left untreated."

Other types of eye cancer (e.g., conjunctival melanoma, orbital tumors).

"Other types of eye cancer include:

- Conjunctival melanoma: This rare cancer develops in the conjunctiva, the thin membrane covering the white part of the eye (sclera). It may appear as a pigmented lesion or a red patch on the eye, and can cause symptoms like blurred vision, eye pain, or sensitivity to light. Conjunctival melanoma is more common in older adults and can spread to the lymph nodes and other parts of the body if left untreated.

- **Orbital tumors:** These cancers develop in the tissues surrounding the eye, such as the eyelids, tear glands, or fat tissue. Orbital tumors can be benign (non-cancerous) or malignant (cancerous). Benign tumors, like hemangiomas or dermoid cysts, are usually slow-growing and may not require treatment. Malignant orbital tumors, like rhabdomyosarcoma or adenoid cystic carcinoma, can be aggressive and require prompt treatment to prevent vision loss and eye loss.

- **Lymphoma:** This cancer develops in the immune system, which can affect the eyes. Ocular lymphoma can occur in the eyelids, conjunctiva, or retina, and may cause symptoms like eye pain, blurred vision, or eye swelling. There are several types of ocular lymphoma, including Hodgkin lymphoma and non-Hodgkin lymphoma.

- Squamous cell carcinoma: This rare cancer develops in the conjunctiva or cornea, the clear layer on the front of the eye. It may appear as a small, raised lesion or a red patch on the eye, and can cause symptoms like eye pain, blurred vision, or sensitivity to light. Squamous cell carcinoma is more common in older adults and can spread to the lymph nodes and other parts of the body if left untreated.

These types of eye cancer are less common than retinoblastoma and uveal melanoma, but it's essential to be aware of their symptoms and seek medical attention if you notice any unusual changes in your eyes. Early detection and treatment can significantly improve outcomes and prevent vision loss or eye loss."

"## Chapter 3: Causes and Risk Factors

Eye cancer, like other cancers, is a complex disease that is influenced by a combination of genetic and environmental factors. While the exact cause of eye cancer is not always known, research has identified several risk factors that increase the likelihood of developing the disease.

Genetic Factors:

- Family history: A family history of eye cancer or other cancers, such as melanoma or retinoblastoma, can increase an individual's risk. This is because certain genetic mutations can be inherited from parents or passed down through generations.

- Inherited genetic syndromes: Certain genetic syndromes, such as retinoblastoma, neurofibromatosis, or familial adenomatous polyposis (FAP), can increase the risk of developing eye cancer. These syndromes are often caused by inherited genetic mutations.

- Genetic mutations: Specific genetic mutations, such as those in the RB1 or TP53 genes, can increase the risk of eye cancer. These mutations can occur spontaneously or be inherited from parents.

Environmental Factors:

- Ultraviolet (UV) radiation: Prolonged exposure to UV radiation from the sun or tanning beds increases the risk of eye cancer. UV radiation can damage the DNA in eye cells, leading to genetic mutations and cancer.

- Smoking: Smoking has been linked to an increased risk of eye cancer, particularly uveal melanoma. Smoking can damage the eyes and increase the risk of genetic mutations.

- Exposure to chemicals: Certain chemicals, such as pesticides (e.g., insecticides or herbicides), solvents (e.g., benzene or trichloroethylene), or heavy metals (e.g., lead or mercury), have been linked to an increased risk of eye cancer. These chemicals can damage eye cells and increase the risk of genetic mutations.

Other Risk Factors:

- Age: The risk of eye cancer increases with age, with most cases occurring in people over 50 years old.

- Race: Certain races, such as Caucasians, are at higher risk of developing eye cancer, particularly uveal melanoma.

- Previous eye diseases: Certain eye diseases, such as cataracts, glaucoma, or retinal detachment, may increase the risk of eye cancer.

Other Risk Factors:_

1. _Previous eye injuries:_ If you've had a serious eye injury in the past, you may be at higher risk of developing eye cancer.

2. _Certain medications:_ Some medications, such as those used to treat autoimmune disorders or organ transplant patients, can increase the risk of eye cancer.

3. _Radiation exposure:_ If you've had radiation therapy to the head

or neck, you may be at higher risk of developing eye cancer.

4. _Fair skin and light eyes:_ People with fair skin and light eyes are more susceptible to the harmful effects of UV radiation, which can increase their risk of eye cancer.

Protecting Your Eyes:

1. _Wear sunglasses:_ Sunglasses with 100% UV protection can help block harmful UV radiation from the sun.

2. _Wear protective eyewear:_ If you work with chemicals or are exposed to radiation, wear protective eyewear to shield your eyes.

3. _Get regular eye exams:_ Regular eye exams can help detect eye cancer early, when it's most treatable.

4. _Avoid smoking and limit alcohol consumption:_ Both smoking and excessive alcohol consumption can increase your risk of eye cancer.

By understanding the causes and risk factors of eye cancer, you can take steps to protect your eyes and reduce your risk of developing this disease. Early detection and treatment are key to preventing vision loss and eye loss, so don't hesitate to seek medical attention if you notice any unusual changes in your eyes.

Chapter 4: Symptoms and Diagnosis,

Symptoms of Eye Cancer

Eye cancer can be asymptomatic in its early stages, but as it progresses, it can cause a range of symptoms, including:

- *Blurred vision or vision loss*: This is one of the most common symptoms of eye cancer, and it can occur in one or both eyes. For example, you may notice that your vision is blurry or fuzzy, or that you have trouble seeing objects clearly.

- *Double vision or eye movement problems*: Eye cancer can cause problems with eye movement, leading to double vision or difficulty moving your eyes. For example, you may notice that your eyes feel weak or tired, or that you have trouble moving your eyes from side to side.

- *Eye pain or discomfort*: Eye cancer can cause pain or discomfort in the eye, which can range from mild to severe. For example, you may feel a sharp pain in your eye, or a dull ache that doesn't go away.

- *Sensitivity to light*: Eye cancer can cause sensitivity to light, which can make it uncomfortable to be outside or in bright lighting. For example, you may need to wear sunglasses indoors or avoid going outside during peak sunlight hours.

- *Redness or swelling of the eye*: Eye cancer can cause redness or swelling of the eye, which can be noticeable and unsightly. For example, your eye may look red or puffy, or you may notice swelling around the eye.

- *Change in eye color or shape*: In some cases, eye cancer can cause a change in eye color or shape. For example, your eye may appear larger or smaller than usual, or the color of your iris may change.

- *Flashes of light or floating objects in vision*: Eye cancer can cause flashes of light or floating objects in vision, which can be alarming and disruptive. For example, you may see flashes of light or floating spots in your vision, even when your eyes are closed.

Diagnosis of Eye Cancer

If you experience any of these symptoms, it's important to see an eye doctor (ophthalmologist or optometrist) right away. They will perform a comprehensive eye exam to determine the cause of your symptoms.

The diagnosis of eye cancer typically involves a combination of the following tests:

- *Visual acuity test*: This test measures your ability to see objects clearly at a distance. For example, you may be asked to read an eye chart or identify objects on a screen.

- *Dilated eye exam*: This test allows your eye doctor to see the inside of your eye more clearly. For example, they may use eye drops to dilate your pupils and then examine your eye with a special magnifying lens.

- *Imaging tests*: Imaging tests like ultrasound, MRI, or CT scans can help your eye doctor see the tumor in your eye. For example, they may use ultrasound to create images of the eye or MRI to create detailed images of the eye and surrounding tissues.

- *Biopsy*: In some cases, a biopsy may be necessary to confirm the diagnosis of eye cancer. For example, your eye doctor may remove a small sample of tissue from your eye and send it to a laboratory for examination.

Highlights

- Eye cancer can be asymptomatic in its early stages, but it can cause a range of symptoms as it progresses.

- Symptoms of eye cancer can include blurred vision, double vision, eye pain, sensitivity to light, redness or swelling of the eye, change in eye color or shape, and flashes of light or floating objects in vision.

- The diagnosis of eye cancer typically involves a combination of visual acuity test, dilated eye exam, imaging tests, and biopsy.

- Early detection and treatment are key to preventing vision loss and eye loss from eye cancer.

Chapter 5: Treatment and Management of Eye Cancer

Treatment for eye cancer depends on the type and severity of the cancer, as well as the patient's overall health. The goal of treatment is to remove the tumor, preserve vision, and prevent the cancer from spreading to other parts of the body.

Surgical Procedures

1. *Enucleation*: Removal of the affected eye
   - Procedure: The surgeon makes an incision in the eye socket,

carefully removes the eye, and closes the socket with stitches.

   - Risks: Infection, bleeding, socket contracture

2. *Evisceration*: Removal of the eye contents, leaving the eye shell intact

   - Procedure: The surgeon makes an incision in the eye, removes the eye contents, and fills the eye with an implant.

   - Risks: Infection, bleeding, implant rejection

3. *Exenteration*: Removal of the eye and surrounding tissues

- Procedure: The surgeon makes an incision in the eye socket, removes the eye and surrounding tissues, and closes the socket with stitches.

- Risks: Infection, bleeding, facial disfigurement

Radiation Therapy

1. *External Beam Radiation*: Radiation is directed at the tumor from outside the body

- Procedure: The patient is positioned on a table, and a machine directs radiation at the tumor.

- Risks: Eye dryness, cataracts, vision loss

2. *Brachytherapy*: Radiation is placed inside the eye, near the tumor

- Procedure: The surgeon implants a small radioactive device in the eye, which is removed after treatment.

- Risks: Infection, bleeding, radiation exposure

Chemotherapy

1. *Systemic Chemotherapy*: Drugs are administered orally or intravenously to kill cancer cells

   - Procedure: The patient takes drugs as directed by their doctor.

   - Risks: Nausea, hair loss, fatigue

2. *Intravitreal Chemotherapy*: Drugs are injected directly into the eye

- Procedure: The surgeon injects drugs into the eye using a small needle.

   - Risks: Infection, bleeding, vision loss

Targeted Therapy

1. *Laser Therapy*: High-energy light is used to kill cancer cells

   - Procedure: The surgeon uses a laser to target and destroy cancer cells.

   - Risks: Eye damage, vision loss

2. *Photodynamic Therapy*: A light-sensitive drug is used to kill cancer cells

   - Procedure: The patient is given a light-sensitive drug, and a special light is used to activate the drug.

   - Risks: Eye damage, vision loss

Risks and Complications

- Infection

- Bleeding

- Vision loss

- Eye dryness

- Cataracts

- Facial disfigurement

- Radiation exposure

- Nausea

- Hair loss

- Fatigue

It's important to note that each patient's treatment plan is unique and may involve a combination of these procedures. It's essential to discuss the potential risks and benefits with a qualified healthcare professional.

Let's break down the risks associated with eye cancer treatment, one by one, with a detailed explanation, possible remedies, and therapies:

Risk 1: Infection

Infection is a potential risk of eye cancer treatment, particularly with surgical procedures. Bacteria can enter the eye through the incision site, leading to infection.

Detailed Explanation: Infection can occur when bacteria enter the eye through the incision site, causing inflammation, redness, and discharge. If left untreated, infection can lead to serious complications, including vision loss and eye loss.

Remedy/Therapy:

- Antibiotics: Administered orally or topically to combat infection

- Antiviral medication: Used to treat viral infections

- Anti-inflammatory medication: Reduces inflammation and swelling

- Wound care: Proper cleaning and dressing of the incision site to prevent infection

Risk 2: Bleeding

Bleeding is a potential risk of eye cancer treatment, particularly with surgical procedures. Bleeding can occur during or after surgery, leading to vision loss and eye damage.

Detailed Explanation: Bleeding can occur due to damage to blood vessels during surgery, leading to hemorrhage. If left untreated, bleeding can lead to vision loss and eye damage.

Remedy/Therapy:

- Cauterization: Applying heat or cold to stop bleeding

- Suturing: Stitches to close bleeding vessels

- Medication: Administered to control bleeding

- Pressure bandage: Applied to the eye to control bleeding

Risk 3: Vision Loss

Vision loss is a potential risk of eye cancer treatment, particularly with surgical procedures. Vision loss can occur due to damage to the optic nerve or retina.

Detailed Explanation: Vision loss can occur due to damage to the optic nerve or retina during surgery, leading to permanent vision loss.

Remedy/Therapy:

- Vision rehabilitation: Training to adapt to vision loss

- Low vision aids: Magnifying glasses or contact lenses to enhance vision

- Orientation and mobility training: Training to navigate with vision loss

- Counseling: Psychological support to cope with vision loss

Risk 4: Eye Dryness

Eye dryness is a potential risk of eye cancer treatment, particularly with radiation therapy. Eye dryness can lead to discomfort and vision problems.

Detailed Explanation: Eye dryness can occur due to radiation damage to the tear glands, leading to reduced tear production.

Remedy/Therapy:

- Artificial tears: Lubricating eye drops to moisturize the eye

- Punctal plugs: Small devices inserted into the tear ducts to block drainage

- Humidifiers: Devices that add moisture to the air

- Warm compresses: Applied to the eyes to stimulate tear production

Risk 5: Cataracts

Cataracts are a potential risk of eye cancer treatment, particularly with radiation therapy. Cataracts can lead to vision loss and blindness.

Detailed Explanation: Cataracts can occur due to radiation damage to the lens, leading to clouding and vision loss.

Remedy/Therapy:

- Cataract surgery: Surgical removal of the cloudy lens

- Intraocular lens implantation: Implantation of an artificial lens

- Glasses or contact lenses: Corrective lenses to improve vision

- Low vision aids: Magnifying glasses or contact lenses to enhance vision

Risk 6: Facial Disfigurement

Facial disfigurement is a potential risk of eye cancer treatment, particularly with exenteration. Facial disfigurement can lead to emotional and psychological distress.

Facial disfigurement can occur due to the removal of the eye and surrounding tissues, leading to a change in facial appearance.

Remedy/Therapy:

- Reconstructive surgery: Surgical reconstruction of the eye socket and surrounding tissues

- Prosthetic eye: A artificial eye that matches the natural eye

- Counseling: Psychological support to cope with facial disfigurement

- Support groups: Connecting with others who have experienced similar disfigurement

Risk 7: Radiation Exposure

Radiation exposure is a potential risk of eye cancer treatment, particularly with radiation therapy. Radiation exposure can lead to secondary cancers and other health problems.

Radiation exposure can occur due to the use of radiation to treat eye cancer, leading to exposure to harmful radiation.

Remedy/Therapy:

- Radiation shielding: Using protective shielding to minimize radiation exposure

- Radiation dosing: Careful calculation of radiation doses to minimize exposure

- Regular check-ups: Monitoring for secondary cancers and other health problems

- Protective gear: Wearing protective gear, such as gloves and masks, to minimize radiation exposure

Risk 8: Nausea and Vomiting

Nausea and vomiting are potential risks of eye cancer treatment, particularly with chemotherapy. Nausea and vomiting can lead to dehydration and malnutrition.

Nausea and vomiting can occur due to the use of chemotherapy drugs, leading to stomach upset and vomiting.

Remedy/Therapy:

- Anti-nausea medication: Administered to alleviate nausea and vomiting

- Hydration therapy: Intravenous fluids to prevent dehydration

- Nutritional support: Ensuring adequate nutrition to prevent malnutrition

- Relaxation techniques: Techniques, such as deep breathing and meditation, to manage nausea and vomiting

Risk 9: Hair Loss

Hair loss is a potential risk of eye cancer treatment, particularly with chemotherapy. Hair loss can lead to emotional distress and changes in appearance.

Detailed Explanation: Hair loss can occur due to the use of chemotherapy drugs, leading to hair thinning or complete hair loss.

Remedy/Therapy:

- Hair loss support: Counseling and support to cope with hair loss

- Wigs and hairpieces: Providing artificial hair to cover hair loss

- Head coverings: Hats, scarves, and other head coverings to conceal hair loss

- Hair growth medication: Medication to stimulate hair growth after chemotherapy

Risk 10: Fatigue

Fatigue is a potential risk of eye cancer treatment, particularly with chemotherapy and radiation therapy. Fatigue can lead to decreased productivity and emotional distress.

Detailed Explanation: Fatigue can occur due to the physical and emotional demands of eye cancer treatment, leading to feelings of exhaustion and tiredness.

Remedy/Therapy:

- Rest and relaxation: Encouraging rest and relaxation to conserve energy

- Energy conservation: Techniques to manage energy levels and conserve energy

- Exercise therapy: Gentle exercise to improve energy levels and overall health

- Support groups: Connecting with others who have experienced similar fatigue

Risk 11: Eye Damage

Eye damage is a potential risk of eye cancer treatment, particularly with radiation therapy and surgery. Eye damage can lead to vision loss and eye pain.

Detailed Explanation: Eye damage can occur due to the use of radiation therapy or surgical procedures, leading to damage to the eye tissues and vision loss.

Remedy/Therapy:

- Vision rehabilitation: Training to adapt to vision loss

- Low vision aids: Magnifying glasses or contact lenses to enhance vision

- Eye pain management: Medication and techniques to manage eye pain

- Regular check-ups: Monitoring for eye damage and vision loss

Risk 12: Secondary Cancers

Secondary cancers are a potential risk of eye cancer treatment, particularly with radiation therapy. Secondary cancers can occur in other parts of the body.

Detailed Explanation: Secondary cancers can occur due to the use of radiation therapy, which can increase the risk of developing cancer in other parts of the body.

Remedy/Therapy:

- Regular check-ups: Monitoring for secondary cancers

- Cancer screening: Regular screening for secondary cancers

- Risk reduction: Avoiding risk factors for secondary cancers

- Support groups: Connecting with others who have experienced secondary cancers

Risk 13: Immune System Suppression

Immune system suppression is a potential risk of eye cancer

treatment, particularly with chemotherapy. Immune system suppression can increase the risk of infections.

Detailed Explanation: Immune system suppression can occur due to the use of chemotherapy drugs, which can weaken the immune system.

Remedy/Therapy:

- Infection prevention: Taking steps to prevent infections

- Antibiotics: Administering antibiotics to treat infections

- Immune system support: Providing support to the immune system

- Regular check-ups: Monitoring for immune system suppression

Risk 14: Emotional Distress

Emotional distress is a potential risk of eye cancer treatment, particularly with facial disfigurement and vision loss. Emotional distress can lead to anxiety and depression.

Detailed Explanation: Emotional distress can occur due to the physical and emotional demands of eye cancer treatment, leading to feelings of anxiety and depression.

Remedy/Therapy:

- Counseling: Providing emotional support and counseling

- Support groups: Connecting with others who have experienced similar emotional distress

- Relaxation techniques: Techniques to manage stress and anxiety

- Medication: Administering medication to manage anxiety and depression

Risk 15: Financial Burden

Financial burden is a potential risk of eye cancer treatment, particularly with the high cost of medical care. Financial burden can lead to stress and anxiety.

Detailed Explanation: Financial burden can occur due to the high cost of eye cancer treatment, including surgery, radiation therapy, and chemotherapy.

Remedy/Therapy:

- Financial assistance: Providing financial assistance and resources

- Insurance support: Helping patients navigate insurance coverage

- Cost transparency: Providing clear information about treatment costs

- Fundraising support: Encouraging fundraising efforts to support patients

Risk 16: Vision Loss

Vision loss is a potential risk of eye cancer treatment, particularly with surgery and radiation therapy. Vision loss can lead to blindness and impaired daily functioning.

Detailed Explanation: Vision loss can occur due to damage to the eye and surrounding tissues during treatment.

Remedy/Therapy:

- Vision rehabilitation: Training to adapt to vision loss

- Low vision aids: Magnifying glasses or contact lenses to enhance vision

- Orientation and mobility training: Training to navigate with vision loss

- Counseling: Emotional support to cope with vision loss

Risk 17: Eye Movement Impairment

Eye movement impairment is a potential risk of eye cancer treatment, particularly with surgery and radiation therapy. Eye movement impairment can lead to difficulty reading, driving, and performing daily tasks.

Detailed Explanation: Eye movement impairment can occur due to damage to the eye muscles and nerves during treatment.

Remedy/Therapy:

- Eye exercises: Exercises to improve eye movement

- Prism lenses: Special lenses to improve eye alignment

- Vision therapy: Training to improve eye movement and vision

- Adaptive equipment: Providing equipment to assist with daily tasks

Risk 18: Corneal Ulceration

Corneal ulceration is a potential risk of eye cancer treatment, particularly with radiation therapy. Corneal ulceration can lead to eye pain, vision loss, and even blindness.

Detailed Explanation: Corneal ulceration can occur due to radiation damage to the cornea, leading to open sores and vision loss.

Remedy/Therapy:

- Topical antibiotics: Medication to treat corneal ulcers

- Pain management: Medication to manage eye pain

- Corneal transplantation: Surgical replacement of the cornea

- Protective shielding: Using protective shielding to minimize radiation exposure

Risk 19: Glaucoma

Glaucoma is a potential risk of eye cancer treatment, particularly with radiation therapy. Glaucoma can lead to vision loss and blindness.

Detailed Explanation: Glaucoma can occur due to radiation damage to the optic nerve, leading to increased eye pressure and vision loss.

Remedy/Therapy:

- Medication: Eye drops or oral medication to reduce eye pressure
- Surgery: Surgical procedures to improve eye drainage

- Laser therapy: Laser treatment to improve eye drainage

- Regular monitoring: Regular check-ups to monitor eye pressure and vision

Risk 20: Eyelid Deformity

Eyelid deformity is a potential risk of eye cancer treatment, particularly with surgery and radiation therapy. Eyelid deformity can lead to eye discomfort and vision problems.

Detailed Explanation: Eyelid deformity can occur due to surgery or radiation damage to the eyelid, leading to drooping or sagging eyelids.

Remedy/Therapy:

- Eyelid surgery: Surgical correction of eyelid deformity

- Eyelid exercises: Exercises to improve eyelid movement

- Eyelid prosthesis: Artificial eyelid to improve appearance

- Supportive care: Providing supportive care to manage eye discomfort

Risk 21: Orbital Bone Damage

Orbital bone damage is a potential risk of eye cancer treatment, particularly with surgery and radiation therapy. Orbital bone damage can lead to eye socket deformity and vision problems.

Detailed Explanation: Orbital bone damage can occur due to surgery or radiation damage to the bones surrounding the eye, leading to deformity and vision problems.

Remedy/Therapy:

- Orbital reconstruction: Surgical reconstruction of the eye socket

- Bone grafting: Transplanting healthy bone tissue to repair damaged bone

- Radiation therapy: Using radiation to shrink tumors and reduce damage

- Supportive care: Providing supportive care to manage eye discomfort

Risk 22: Optic Nerve Damage

Optic nerve damage is a potential risk of eye cancer treatment, particularly with radiation therapy. Optic nerve damage can lead to vision loss and blindness.

Detailed Explanation: Optic nerve damage can occur due to radiation damage to the optic nerve, leading to vision loss and blindness.

Remedy/Therapy:

- Radiation shielding: Using protective shielding to minimize radiation exposure

- Optic nerve repair: Surgical repair of damaged optic nerve

- Vision rehabilitation: Training to adapt to vision loss

- Supportive care: Providing supportive care to manage vision loss

Risk 23: Eye Muscle Damage

Eye muscle damage is a potential risk of eye cancer treatment, particularly with surgery and radiation therapy. Eye muscle damage can lead to eye movement impairment and vision problems.

Detailed Explanation: Eye muscle damage can occur due to surgery or radiation damage to the eye muscles, leading to eye movement impairment and vision problems.

Remedy/Therapy:

- Eye exercises: Exercises to improve eye movement

- Prism lenses: Special lenses to improve eye alignment

- Vision therapy: Training to improve eye movement and vision

- Supportive care: Providing supportive care to manage eye discomfort

Risk 24: Cataract Formation

Cataract formation is a potential risk of eye cancer treatment, particularly with radiation therapy. Cataract formation can lead to vision loss and blindness.

Detailed Explanation: Cataract formation can occur due to radiation damage to the lens, leading to clouding and vision loss.

Remedy/Therapy:

- Cataract surgery: Surgical removal of the cloudy lens

- Intraocular lens implantation: Implantation of an artificial lens

- Vision rehabilitation: Training to adapt to vision loss

- Supportive care: Providing supportive care to manage vision loss

Risk 25: Glaucoma Relapse

Glaucoma relapse is a potential risk of eye cancer treatment, particularly with radiation therapy.

Glaucoma relapse can lead to vision loss and blindness.

Detailed Explanation: Glaucoma relapse can occur due to radiation damage to the optic nerve, leading to increased eye pressure and vision loss.

Remedy/Therapy:

- Medication: Eye drops or oral medication to reduce eye pressure

- Surgery: Surgical procedures to improve eye drainage

- Laser therapy: Laser treatment to improve eye drainage

- Regular monitoring: Regular check-ups to monitor eye pressure and vision

Please note that this list is not exhaustive, and it's essential to consult a healthcare professional for personalized information and guidance on eye cancer treatment risks and remedies.

Chapter 6: Rehabilitation and Support

Rehabilitation and support are crucial aspects of eye cancer treatment. The goal of rehabilitation is to help patients adapt to any physical or visual changes caused by the treatment, while support services aim to address emotional and psychological needs.

6.1 Rehabilitation

- Physical rehabilitation: Helps patients regain strength and mobility in the affected eye and surrounding tissues.

- Vision rehabilitation: Trains patients to adapt to vision loss or changes, improving daily functioning.

- Occupational therapy: Assists patients in adapting to new ways of performing daily tasks.

6.2 Support Services

- Counseling: Provides emotional support and guidance to patients and their families.

- Support groups: Connects patients with others who have experienced similar challenges.

- Psychological therapy: Addresses anxiety, depression, and other mental health concerns.

- Social support: Offers practical help with daily tasks and errands.

6.3 Follow-up Care

- Regular check-ups: Monitor patients' progress, address concerns, and adjust treatment plans as needed.

- Imaging tests: Conduct regular imaging tests to detect any recurrences or metastases.

By combining rehabilitation, support services, and follow-up care, patients can receive comprehensive care that addresses their physical, emotional, and psychological needs, enhancing their overall well-being and quality of life.

Chapter 7: Emerging Trends and Future Directions in Eye Cancer Treatment

Eye cancer treatment is a rapidly evolving field, with scientists and researchers continually exploring new technologies and techniques to improve patient outcomes. Some of the emerging trends and future directions in eye cancer treatment include:

7.1 Immunotherapy: Harnessing the Power of the Immune System

Immunotherapy is a type of treatment that uses the body's own immune system to fight cancer. This approach has shown promising results in treating eye melanoma, the most common type of eye cancer. Immunotherapy works by stimulating the immune system to recognize and attack cancer cells, reducing the risk of recurrence and improving overall survival rates.

7.2 Gene Therapy: Repairing Damaged Genes to Prevent Cancer Growth

Gene therapy is a revolutionary approach that involves replacing or repairing damaged genes to prevent cancer growth. This technique has the potential to be a game-changer in the treatment of eye cancer, as it can target the root cause of the disease. Gene therapy can be used to restore normal cellular function, preventing cancer cells from growing and dividing.

7.3 Nanoparticle-Based Treatments: Delivering Drugs Directly to Tumors

Nanoparticle-based treatments involve using tiny particles to deliver drugs directly to tumors. This approach has several advantages, including reducing side effects and improving efficacy. Nanoparticles can be designed to target specific cells or tissues, ensuring that the drug is delivered exactly where it is needed.

7.4 Advanced Radiation Techniques: Stereotactic Body Radiation Therapy (SBRT) and Proton Therapy

Advanced radiation techniques, such as SBRT and proton therapy, offer more precise and effective ways to deliver radiation to tumors. SBRT uses high doses of radiation to destroy tumors in a few fractions, while proton therapy uses protons instead of X-rays to reduce damage to surrounding tissues.

7.5 Personalized Medicine: Tailoring Treatment to Individual Patients' Needs

Personalized medicine involves tailoring treatment to individual patients' needs and genetic profiles. This approach can improve treatment outcomes and reduce side effects by ensuring that patients receive the most effective treatment for their specific type of eye cancer.

7.6 Combination Therapies: Combining Different Treatment Modalities for Enhanced Effectiveness

Combination therapies involve combining different treatment modalities, such as surgery, radiation, and chemotherapy, to achieve better outcomes. This approach can improve treatment outcomes by targeting different aspects of the disease and reducing the risk of recurrence.

These emerging trends and future directions offer hope for even more effective and targeted treatments for eye cancer, improving patient outcomes and quality of life. As research continues to advance, we can expect to see even more innovative approaches to treating this disease.

Chapter 8: Living with Eye Cancer: Navigating the Physical, Emotional, and Psychological Challenges

Living with eye cancer can be a complex and multifaceted experience, affecting not only the physical body but also the emotional and psychological well-being of patients and their loved ones. This chapter delves into the various challenges that arise during this journey and explores coping strategies, rehabilitation techniques, and quality of life considerations.

8.1 Physical Challenges: Managing Symptoms and Side Effects

Eye cancer treatment can result in various physical challenges, including:

- Vision loss or changes: Patients may experience blurred vision, double vision, or loss of peripheral vision.

- Eye pain or discomfort: Pain, itching, or burning sensations in the eye can occur.

- Dry eye or tearing: Changes in tear production can lead to dryness or excessive tearing.

- Sensitivity to light: Patients may experience discomfort or pain when exposed to light.

- Appearance changes: The eye or eyelid may appear different due to surgery or radiation.

8.2 Emotional and Psychological Challenges: Coping with the Emotional Toll

The diagnosis and treatment of eye cancer can also lead to emotional and psychological challenges, including:

- Anxiety and depression: Patients may experience fear, worry, or sadness.

- Fear and uncertainty: Concerns about the future and treatment outcomes can create anxiety.

- Grief and loss: Patients may mourn the loss of their previous life or vision.

- Body image concerns: Changes in appearance can affect self-esteem.

- Relationship changes: Patients may experience shifts in relationships with family and friends.

8.3 Coping Strategies: Finding Strength and Support

To navigate these challenges, patients can employ various coping strategies, including:

- Seeking support from family, friends, and support groups.

- Practicing self-care and stress reduction techniques, such as meditation or yoga.

- Staying informed and educated about the disease.

- Connecting with others who have experienced eye cancer.

- Finding ways to express emotions and feelings through creative outlets or therapy.

8.4 Rehabilitation and Adaptive Techniques: Maximizing Function and Independence

Rehabilitation and adaptive techniques can help patients adapt to vision changes and maintain independence, including:

- Vision rehabilitation therapy.
- Adaptive equipment and technology.
- Orientation and mobility training.
- Counseling and therapy.

8.5 Quality of Life: Prioritizing Well-being and Fulfillment

Despite the challenges, patients can prioritize their quality of life by:

- Prioritizing physical and emotional well-being.

- Engaging in activities that bring joy and fulfillment.

- Celebrating milestones and accomplishments.

- Finding ways to give back and support others.

- Embracing the present moment and looking to the future with hope.

By acknowledging and addressing the physical, emotional, and psychological challenges associated with eye cancer, patients can find ways to navigate their journey with resilience, hope, and courage.

Chapter 9: Conclusion and Future Perspectives

Eye cancer is a rare but potentially life-threatening disease that requires prompt and appropriate treatment. The management of eye cancer has evolved significantly over the years, with various treatment options available depending on the type and stage of the disease.

In this book, we have discussed the various aspects of eye cancer, including its definition, types, causes, symptoms, diagnosis, treatment options, and rehabilitation. We have also explored the emerging trends and future directions in eye cancer treatment, including immunotherapy, gene therapy, nanoparticle-based treatments, advanced radiation techniques, personalized medicine, and combination therapies.

As we look to the future, it is essential to continue researching and developing new and innovative treatments for eye cancer. Some potential areas of focus include:

- Developing more targeted and effective treatments with fewer side effects

- Improving early detection and diagnosis to improve treatment outcomes

- Enhancing patient quality of life through rehabilitation and support services

- Exploring new technologies and techniques, such as artificial intelligence and robotics, to improve treatment precision and accuracy

By working together, we can continue to advance our understanding of eye cancer and develop new and innovative treatments to improve patient outcomes and quality of life.

Appendix:

Additional Resources for Patients and Caregivers

1. Eye Cancer Organizations:

- Eye Cancer Foundation (ECF)
- International Eye Cancer Consortium (IECC)

- Ocular Melanoma Foundation (OMF)

2. Support Groups:

   - Online forums and discussion boards (e.g., Eye Cancer Forum, OMF Support Group)

   - Local support groups (check with hospitals or eye cancer organizations)

3. Rehabilitation and Adaptive Services:

   - Vision rehabilitation therapy programs

   - Adaptive equipment and technology providers

- Orientation and mobility training services

4. Mental Health Resources:

    - Counseling services (individual and group)

    - Online therapy platforms (e.g., BetterHelp, Talkspace)

    - Support hotlines (e.g., National Suicide Prevention Lifeline)

5. Educational Materials:

    - Eye cancer books and e-books

    - Online articles and blogs (e.g., Eye Cancer Forum, OMF Blog)

    - Educational videos and webinars (e.g., ECF Webinars, IECC Videos)

6. Advocacy and Awareness:

   - Eye cancer awareness events (e.g., Eye Cancer Awareness Month)

   - Advocacy organizations (e.g., National Coalition for Vision Health)

7. Online Communities:

   - Social media groups (e.g., Eye Cancer Support Group on Facebook)

   - Online forums and discussion boards (e.g., Reddit's r/eyecancer)

Remember, this appendix is not exhaustive, and resources may vary depending on your location and specific needs. Always consult with your healthcare team for personalized recommendations and support.

- Glossary of terms

1. *Anaplastic*: Refers to cancer cells that are abnormal and grow rapidly.

2. *Benign*: A non-cancerous tumor or growth.

3. *Biopsy*: A procedure to remove a small sample of tissue for examination.

4. *Choroid*: The layer of blood vessels between the sclera and retina.

5. *Enucleation*: Surgical removal of the eye.

6. *External beam radiation*: A type of radiation therapy that directs rays to the tumor from outside the body.

7. *Eye melanoma*: A type of cancer that develops in the eye, often in the choroid or iris.

8. *Iris*: The colored part of the eye.

9. *Macula*: The part of the retina responsible for central vision.

10. *Malignant*: Cancerous.

Here are the explanations for the next 10 terms, listed according to their corresponding numbers:

11. _Adjuvant therapy_: Additional treatment used to supplement primary treatment, aimed at reducing the risk of cancer recurrence.

12. _Angiogenesis_: The formation of new blood vessels, which can feed tumor growth and promote cancer development.

13. _Asymptomatic_: Showing no symptoms, even if cancer is present, making regular check-ups crucial for early detection.

14. _Brachytherapy_: Internal radiation therapy using implants, which deliver radiation directly to the tumor site.

15. _Cancer staging_: Determining the extent and spread of cancer, crucial for developing an effective treatment plan.

16. _Chemotherapy_: Using drugs to kill cancer cells, which can be administered orally or intravenously.

17. _Choroidal melanoma_: A type of eye melanoma affecting the choroid, the layer of blood vessels between the sclera and retina.

18. _Ciliary body melanoma_: A rare type of eye melanoma affecting the ciliary body, responsible for producing the aqueous humor.

19. _Conjunctiva_: The thin membrane covering the white part of the eye, susceptible to cancerous growths.

20. _Cornea_: The transparent front layer of the eye, responsible for refracting light and maintaining vision clarity.

We hope this book has provided a comprehensive and informative resource for patients, caregivers, and healthcare professionals alike.

Together, we can make a difference in the lives of those affected by eye cancer.

www.ingramcontent.com/pod-product-compliance
Lightning Source LLC
Chambersburg PA
CBHW071932210526
45479CB00002B/648